SICK of SICK

HEALTHY HINTS from *Heaven*

Cheryall Sparks, R.N.

TO CONTACT THE AUTHOR

Healthy Hints from Heaven, LLC

P.O. Box 270834 | Houston, TX 77277 | 832.781.8174

info@healthyhintsfromheaven.com

DEDICATION

I dedicate this book to the memory of my beautiful mother and best friend, Vera M. Rhodes.

Because of you, I became a nurse. Thanks for teaching me how to pray and enjoy life!

MY PRAYER

Everyone who reads this book
will become committed to living
a life of health and wellness.

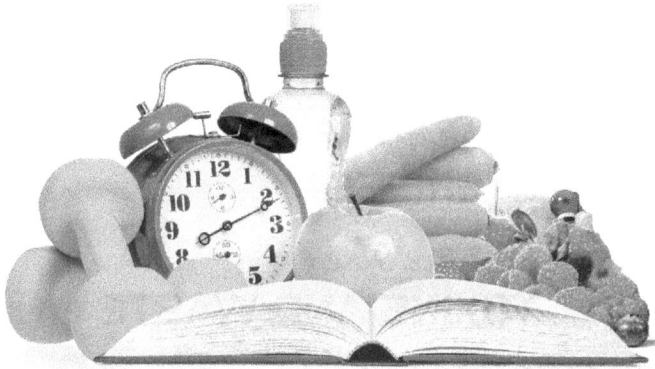

CONTENTS

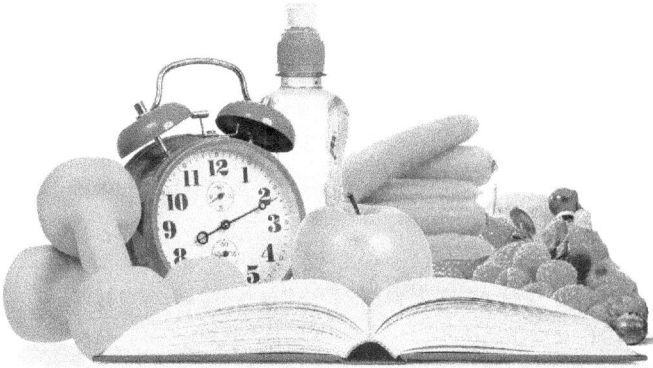

Foreword by

PASTOR JOHN BOWMAN

*H*ealthy Hints from Heaven* provides practical and biblically based truths to assist people in using wisdom for living a healthy lifestyle. Over the years, I have prayed with numerous people seeking healing for things that could have been prevented through following the advice that Cheryall Sparks provides in this straight-forward, no-nonsense book. God can heal you of your diseases, but I believe He also gives us knowledge and understanding so we can live the abundant life He intended for us to live. This is what God desires for each of us:

> **"With long life I will satisfy him**
> **and show him my salvation."**
>
> **—Psalm 91:16**

I have personally seen my body, my health, my energy level, and even my internal peace and joy increase as I have put these "hints" into practice. It takes determination. It is well worth it.

I began with simple things such as intentionally drinking more water. Over time I have been able to add more of these tips to my weekly activities. When I do the right things as prescribed in this book, I feel better inside and out.

Don't settle for less than God's best. Use this book as a guide to health and wholeness. Cheryall starts with what God's Word says and how to have the right belief system. I encourage you to begin daily declaring the powerful scriptures she has provided.

Finally, trust the process. Going from sick to healthy doesn't happen overnight. It may be hard at first, but anything worthwhile comes at a cost. After salvation, there is nothing more valuable than your health. When people are sick they would pay anything to get well. The investment of your time and effort will produce a rewarding payoff—"long life."

—Pastor John Bowman

Senior Director: Men, Singles, Interns, Lay Leaders & LIfegroups

Lakewood Church | Houston, TX

---

*"Worship the Lord Your
God, and His blessing will
be on your food and water.
I will take away sickness
from among you."*

Exodus 23:25 NIV

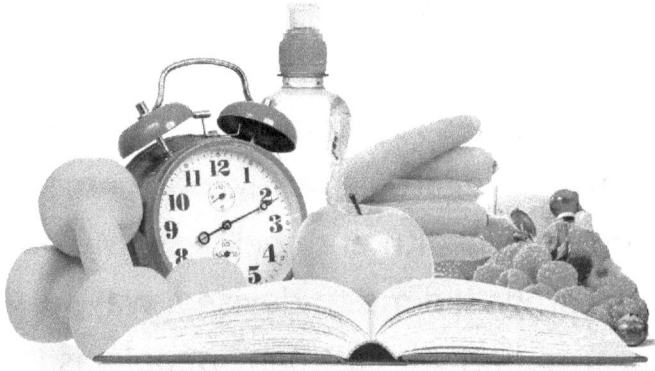

Introduction

WHY I CARE

I am a Registered Nurse with more than 30 years of experience. I am not here to dazzle you with statistics, complicated anatomy, or mysterious disease processes. I am just sick of sick. Throughout my career I have nursed thousands of ill, broken, wounded, and injured people. Every time someone completely recovered, it brought me great joy.

I have learned a tremendous amount of information regarding preventive measures that promote health and wellness. My passion for this compelled me to devise a way to share this information with as many people as I can. I believe that God wants you to flourish in every area of your life. Health and wellness is one of them. I want to help you be able to prevent disease and sickness in your life.

God wants you to *flourish* in *every* area of your life.

At one time, because of my high-stress, sedentary lifestyle and poor eating habits, I was at high risk for diabetes, hypertension, and heart disease. I worked close to twelve hours a day. The few times I would exercise, I went straight to my neighborhood hamburger or fried chicken joint, afterwards. I also loved eating sweets ... I believed dessert should be eaten first!

The demands of my work schedule on top of caring for my own needs meant I never managed to get enough sleep—I never felt truly rested. I remember driving to school one day, getting out of my car, and leaving the car running ... and the car was still moving! I am glad to report **I am no longer living that kind of life.**

Healthy Hints from Heaven allows me to share with you simple things I have learned that are easy to apply which will help you achieve a lifestyle of health and wellness. These hints have helped me arrive at where I am today. As you read this book, please know that I am cheering you on as you become empowered to live a life of health and wellness.

"I will never forget Your commandments, for You have used them to restore my joy and health."

Psalm 119:93 NLT

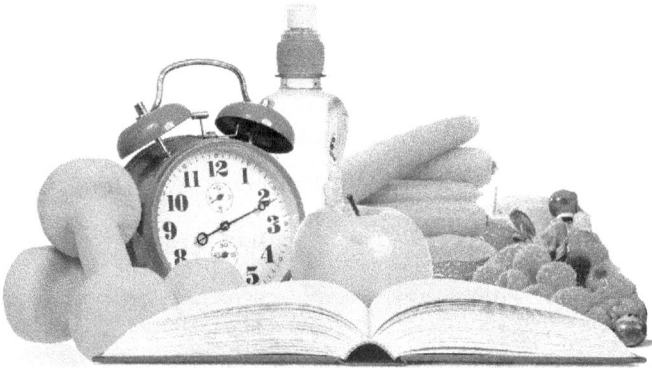

Chapter One

WHAT DO YOU BELIEVE?

BELIEVE: *to accept, trust fully, and in faith, to have a firm conviction as to the reality or goodness of something. To consider to be true and honest.*[1]

1. "believe." Merriam-Webster.com. 2011. http://www.merriamwebster.com (Retrieved December 2014).

*W*hat we believe affects what we do. Our actions and our decisions come from our core—what we believe. Our beliefs become our actions, our actions become our habits, our habits determine our future.

Our belief systems dictate the way we live. They are either the launching pad in fulfilling our God-given destiny, or the anchor that holds us down. When I see sick people I see BONDAGE.

What do you believe about health and wellness?

Do you expect to be healthy and well or do you anticipate sickness and disease? According to the scriptures, God is in favor of our being healthy and well.

> *"... who pardons all your iniquities,*
> *who heals all your diseases."*
> Psalm 103:3 ASV

"... For I will restore health to you and heal all your wounds, says the Lord."

Jeremiah 30:17 AMP

"My son, attend to my words; consent and submit to my sayings. Let them not depart from your spirit; Keep them in the center of your heart. For they are life to those who find them, healing and health to all their flesh."

Proverbs 4:20-22 AMP

"Beloved, I pray that you may prosper in every way and that your body may keep well, even as I know your soul keeps well and prospers."

3 John 2 AMP

I believe our belief system directly affects our health and wellness. Anyone who recovers from sickness and disease does so because of their strong belief system. Start believing what

God says about health and wellness. Let these scriptures settle down in your spirit. Meditate on them. They will shape your thoughts.

As we begin this journey, knowing what God desires for you and what His Word has provided for you will become a part of your belief system. It starts right now. Look at yourself in the mirror and say, "I can live healthy. I can live well."

Even if you are currently experiencing sickness or disease, please know that a life of health and wellness is possible for you. You don't have to stay sick. You don't have to resign yourself to prescriptions and medications for the rest of your life. God has a plan for your body to be completely whole and restored. In fact, He designed your body to heal itself when it is out of balance and to protect itself from things that

A life of *health* and *wellness* is possible for *you!*

attack our cells and break down our immune system.

As a nurse I have spent a lifetime helping sick people feel better. On occasion I have worked with health care professionals that treated only the symptoms and never address the root problems that have caused the sickness in the first place. I have seen a lot of hopelessness and frustration. I have also seen God work in my own life to teach me a better way and show me how He meant for my body to function.

Heaven has a perfect design. All we have to do is cooperate with the *Healthy Hints from Heaven* and stop giving in to the destructive habits and patterns handed to us by the enemy of our soul who WANTS us to be sick!

Are you ready to be well? Are you ready to be healthy? ... then read on!

"The LORD will guide you continually, watering your life when you are dry and keeping you healthy, too. You will be like a well-watered garden, like an ever-flowing spring."

Isaiah 58:11 NLT

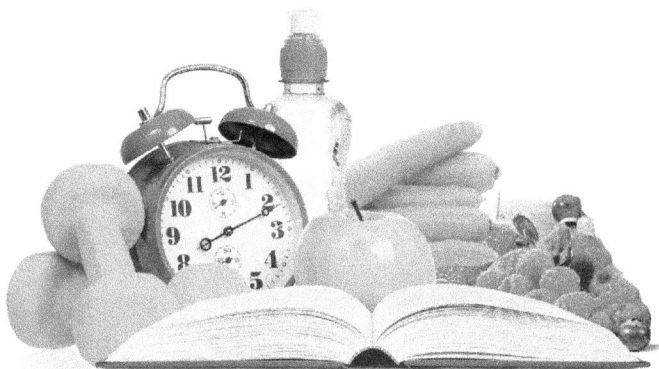

Chapter Two

NOURISHMENT

"God said, 'See, I have given you every plant yielding seed that is on the face of the earth, and every tree with seed in its fruits, You should have for food.'"

Genesis 1:29 AMP

God has provided mankind with all he needs to build his body and sustain life. Man was created with the capacity to live in a state of maximum health and wellness. God intends for us to live a life full of energy, vitality, and vigor. One way He set out for us to accomplish this was to provide us with seeds, nuts, fruits, vegetables, and spices.

Seeds

In its natural state, seeds are composed of proteins, carbohydrates, and fats. They are easy to digest. From seeds we get trees, plants, fruits and vegetables. This lets us know that seeds are filled with the essence of life. You need to eat only a small amount of this concentrated food. According to Dr. N.U. Walker, DSC of *Vegetarian Guide to Diet and Salad*, all seeds and their spirits are among the richest sources of protein, and also rich in calcium and magnesium.

Seeds help give our bodies energy to function properly. They are a great source of dietary fiber which slows down the rate of digestion and helps promote regular bowels. Seeds also help reduce inflammation and according to the Linus Pauling Institute, can reduce your risk of heart disease.[1]

Try to eat some type of seed every day. For the highest nutritional benefits, try eating raw seeds before they have been roasted or salted. Seeds such as pumpkin, sunflower, sesame, and alfalfa are delicious and can be eaten alone or in salads. Some other seeds you may like to try include chia, flax, or hemp seeds.

Pictured here are sesame, flax, pumpkin, and sunflower seeds.

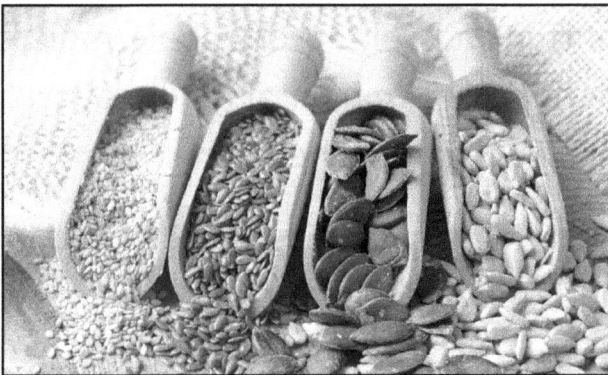

1. "What Are the Health Benefits of Eating Nuts & Seeds" SFGate http:// healthyeating.sfgate.com/health-benefits-eating-nuts-seeds-6701.html (Retrieved May 2015.)

Nuts

Nuts have a very high concentration of protein and fats. They are valuable as nourishment for the bones. When eaten raw, they will supply a burst of energy. They make good in between meal snacks and, like seeds, are also high in fiber.

Some people stay away from nuts, worried that they are fattening, but the truth is eating nuts boosts your intake of healthy, unsaturated fatty acids. The Mayo Clinic advises that nuts can actually lower the "bad" LDL cholesterol levels in your blood. So feel free to sprinkle nuts on your salads or on top of yogurt. Try grinding them into butter and spread on whole grain bread. When shopping, look for almonds, pecans, pine nuts, walnuts, and cashews.

Nuts are high in calories, so keep in mind that a handful goes a long way—proof that good things really do come in small packages!

Herbs and Spices

Herbs and spices are filled with nutrients that promote health and wellness. Some, such as cinnamon, rosemary, cloves, and parsley have antioxidant qualities. Antioxidants help protect our bodies from harmful free radicals which cause damage to cells, impair our immune systems, and can lead to things like heart disease and cancer. Free radicals come from our exposure to toxins, pollution, chemicals, etc.

Some herbs like cayenne and garlic have germ fighting qualities. Ginger and rosemary possess anti-inflammatory properties. Our hair, nails, and teeth can benefit from sage and cloves. Garlic and green tea help strengthen our immune system. There has even been a recent discovery that cinnamon helps to control blood sugar. If you are eating something sweet, try adding a half teaspoon of cinnamon to it.

Other herbs and spices keep our joints functioning properly. These includes turmeric, parsley, oregano, and mint. Eat these fresh. Cook with them. Know that you are giving your body much needed nutrients and protection from disease.

Herbs and spices add more than flavor ... they help keep you healthy!

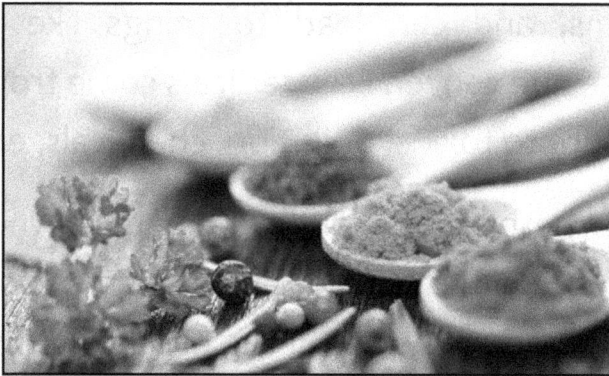

Fruits and Vegetables

Eating fruits and vegetables are another way to replenish life to our bodies. We are blessed to live in a country where they are so plentiful. Organically grown fruits and vegetables are highly recommended. If you buy those grown commercially, remember to wash them with a vegetable brush and use a veggie and fruit wash. Also, it is best to let them soak in water for about 10 minutes.

You may eat them fresh and raw, steamed, sautéed, roasted, or slow cooked—as long as you eat them! Researchers feel that a number of vegetables and fruits also have antioxidants. This reduces the risk of heart disease, cancer, and diabetes. Some examples of those high in antioxidants are apples, blueberries, carrots, spinach, and broccoli. These help cleanse the body and can contain proteins and carbohydrates. Most are available frozen or even bottled or canned as juices when fresh is not a possibility for you.

Be sure to include fruits and vegetables in your daily meals or as snacks. I encourage you to experiement with some you might be unfamiliar with. You may be surprised at how good they taste! Some examples of these healthy jewels are beets, cabbage, cucumbers, blackberries, cranberries, plums, oranges, cauliflower, lettuce, asparagus and squash.

I eat at least four servings a day. If you are just starting out, begin by trying to incorporate one serving in one meal at a time. Every tiny good decision you make takes you in the direction of better health. Don't be discouraged if you are overweight or battling disease. Don't give in. Even eating just one piece of fresh fruit a day as a replacement for a cookie or treat will begin to have positive benefits for your health.

Over time I began to also eat salads every day. I mix kale, lettuce, tomatoes, cucumbers, carrots, and red onions together. I use dressings sparingly as this takes away from the taste of the salad. This "salad habit" has kept me searching for new vegetables and fruits to place in my salads. I recently began to eat papaya and I am looking forward to tasting durian (a small tropical fruit native to Malaysia). I receive much energy and vitality from eating fruits and vegetables ... and you can too!

Proteins

Proteins are like the Legos®—the essential building blocks of the body.[1] All proteins are made up of amino acids. Just like Legos®, combinations of amino acids build together to form proteins.

Proteins provide our bodies with energy. Though many people think of meat, fish, poultry, and dairy products as the main source of protein, you can obtain protein a number of ways. Many nuts, seeds, and vegetables give the body exactly what it needs—the amino acids required—to build protein.

Even when you eat a food that is considered "protein" (like meat), your body first has to break that protein down into amino acids before it can be used in the body as fuel. This is why I encourage you to think beyond the meat counter when planning how to have enough protien in your body for healthy muscles and energy. To

---

1.   *The Great Physician RX for Health and Wellness.* © 2005. Jordan Rubin, MD; David Remedios, MD. pg. 19.

receive the maximum nutritional value from these sources, look for them in their healthiest form. Your intake of protein is totally up to you. It is a matter of personal taste, preference, and judgment. Let balance and moderation guide your decisions.

Water

The value to your body from drinking water is great—much more than I can share with you here. The average person's body is composed of approximately 60-70% water. It is a known fact that we can survive without food—up to 40 days—but without water, life would end in approximately 3 to 5 days. Water helps move nutrients throughout our bodies. It keeps our lungs lubricated and moist, making breathing easier. It removes waste from our cells and helps maintain normal body temperature.

We continually lose water through sweating and elimination, so it has to be continuously replenished. We must drink water even when we do not feel thirsty.

When I finally grasped this important concept, I started adding lemons and sipping water throughout the day. The lemon helped give water a "taste" and I was surprised! I realized that I drank close to four glasses of water by the end of that day!

Here are just a few of the benefits you receive from drinking water.

- Drinking water can help you control the amount of calories you eat ... and drink! Imagine how many calories you would save by replacing 32 oz. of a sugary, carbonated beverage with 32 oz. of clear, pure, healthy water!

- Drinking water helps energize your muscles. This is especially important for exercising. If you have not had enough water your muscles will quickly become fatigued and you will have little to no endurance.

- Drinking water helps your skin stay clear and healthy. In fact, dehydration makes lines and wrinkles deeper and more noticeable. Hydration is a beauty secret!

- Drinking enough water helps with healthy digestion, allowing your body to absorb the nutrients you ate and flush waste from your system through healthy kidneys and a hydrated intestinal tract.

Water is in abundant supply, so start drinking! Most sources advocate 6 - 8 glasses of water each day and I completely agree! I encourage you to drink the highest quality of water you can. Clean water is able to carry out its functions at the maximum level. Bottled water and water purifiers can help you achieve this. If you are having difficulty drinking water, I suggest you pray to our Heavenly Father, God. He will help you to drink more water.

More Healthy Hints

- **Eat breakfast.** Breakfast is important because it jump starts your ability to burn calories at the beginning of the day.

- **Shop smart.** Shop the outer perimeter of your grocery store for the healthiest options—fresh produce, fresh meats, fresh dairy. Limit the middle aisles where all the canned and processed foods are offered.

- **Eat less more often.** Eating small amounts of nutritious meals every three to four hours will keep you from feeling hungry.

- **Chew your meal slowly.** This allows you to taste your food and enjoy it. It helps prevent over-eating and makes sure what you swallow is already breaking down. (Your body has to work harder to digest when you gulp down your food!)

- **Read labels**. The fewer ingredients listed, the more authentic and less processed the product is likely to be.

- **Know when to quit**. Eat only until you feel satisfied, not until you are full.

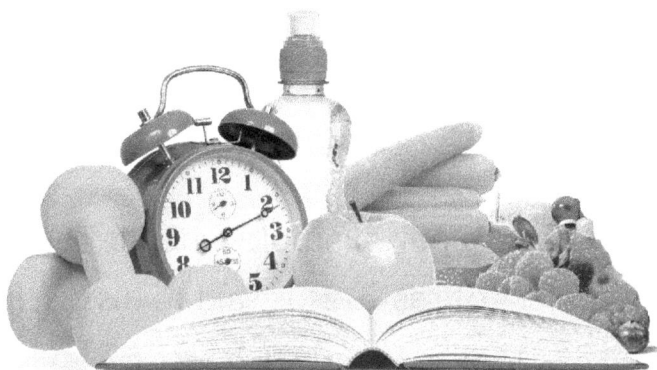

Chapter Three

REST AND SLEEP

"Come to Me, all you who labor and are heavy-laden and overburdened, and I will cause you to rest. I will ease and relieve and refresh your souls.

Matthew 11:28 AMP

Rest

*J*esus Christ is our example when it comes to the subject of rest. Jesus said to his disciples:

"Come away by yourselves, to a deserted place and rest awhile."

Mark 6:31 AMP

The essence of this comment was to disconnect from all of the mental, emotional and physical things that drain us of life. A "deserted" place means a place free from life's many distractions. This includes social media, cell phones, computers, iPads, televisions, etc. A "deserted" place is quiet and peaceful. It is a place that allows when you get alone, to be able to focus on God.

God is the source of rest and restoration.

God is the source of rest and restoration. So the goal is to find at least 10 or 15 minutes of time where you pull away from all distractions and spend that time alone with God. Try to do this every day. As you make this a priority, you will be surprised how this time will begin to expand. Show God that you are committed to seeking and spending time with Him and in turn, He will make your days prosperous.

At one point in my life, I was working and going to school. This meant I was committed 60-70 hours a week ... not to mention drive time! One evening I began to experience a severe headache. It was so severe I could hardly stand upright. Somehow, I managed to drive myself home, but my headache only intensified. I called my parents, and my father took me to the local emergency room where a doctor walked into my room and asked me one question: "What is your priority?"

The question stunned me. This is not what most doctors ask when seeking your medical history. I thought for a moment and realized I was chasing the American dream at the expense of my health. I knew that I had to make some serious changes.

The nurse came and administered medicine that got rid of the headache. When I arrived back at home, I knew I had to answer that question: "What was my priority?" My lifestyle did not reflect my heart—the answer was God.

So, I began to change how I spent my time and started spending more time with Him. I spent time in prayer, in praise, and reading my Bible. I spent just 10 minutes at first, and it grew from there. Now, I am blessed to have a job where I get an extra day off. Many times I take a day and spend it resting and connecting with God. When I return to the "real world" I tackle life's problems from a position of rest.

I tackle life's *problems* from a *position* of *rest*.

I am much more creative, efficient, and productive. At the end of my day I feel a sense of satisfaction and accomplishment. Every day is not perfect, but I know that I have the victory because of my time of rest with God. Start today. Start with 10 minutes and watch it grow. Your life will change for the better.

Sleep

"For He giveth His beloved sleep ..."

Psalms 127:2 KJV

Sleep is a necessity of life. God gives us sleep. A good night's sleep revitalizes our weary and fatigued bodies. Sleep allows our bodies to be restored. It prepares us for a creative, purposeful, and productive day. Science has revealed that during periods of sleep, our bodies are rebuilt—our cells are literally renewed.

During sleep, our bodies go through a cleansing process. Dr. Richard Bootzin at the University Of Arizona Sleep Disorder Center discovered that people who got 7 to 8 hours of sleep each night lived longer, happier, and healthier lives.[1] How can you measure whether you are getting an adequate amount of sleep? Ask yourself these questions:

- Do I wake up easily?

- Do I feel energetic when I awake?

- Do I have an entire day of creativity and productivity?

If the answer is yes, then you are getting enough sleep whether it is 5 hours or 8 hours. Individual requirements for sleep vary, and your own requirements will change in different seasons of your life. The important point is that every human being needs sleep to be able to function at their best. Most of us do not think about our sleeping habits or take time to adjust or enhance our sleep

---

1.   *Prescription for Natural Healing.* Avery Publishers. © 2000. Phyllis A. Balch, CNC. Pg. 476.

patterns. If you want to receive the fullest benefit from sleep, try the following:

- Pray before going to sleep.

- Read a chapter of the Bible before sleeping.

- Go to bed at the same time every night.

- Use your bedroom only for sleep.

More Healthy Hints

· **Eat light meals in the evening**. This gives the digestive system a chance to rest.

· **Eat foods that promote sleep**. Drink milk, eat bananas, dates, and yogurt.

· **Prepare your bedroom for sleep**. Make it comfortable with restful sounds such as falling rain or ocean waves.

---

*"In peace I will lie down
and sleep, for you alone, O
LORD, will keep me safe."*

Psalm 4:8 NLT

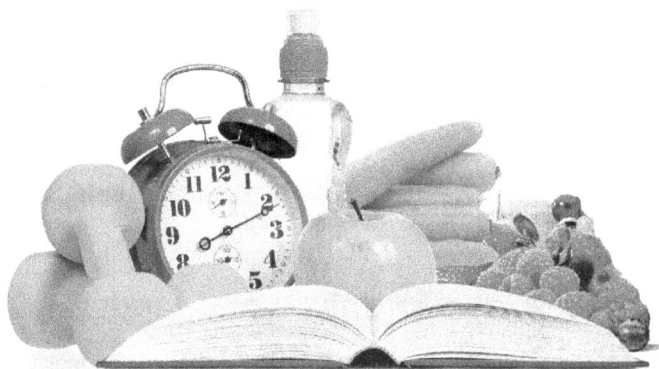

Chapter Four

EXERCISE

"For the moment all discipline seems painful rather than pleasant, but later it yields the peaceful fruit of righteousness to those who have been trained by it. Therefore lift up your drooping hands and strengthen your weak knees ..."

Hebrews 12:11-12 ESV

---

*R*egular exercise improves digestion, circulation, and elimination. It increases our energy levels. It reduces stress and anxiety. It increases our strength and endurance. It doesn't really matter what you choose as long as you make some type of physical activity part of a regular habit. The key is to do it consistently. You can join a gym, purchase used gym equipment to use at home, or just walk around your neighborhood, school, or park. It does not have to be expensive. Other suggestions:

Water Aerobics

- Cycling

- Jogging

- Swimming

- Sit-ups/Pushups

- Playing Sports (Football, Volleyball, etc.)

To receive the maximum benefit from exercise you must be consistent and diligent. Try to exercise three to four times a week. Select an exercise that you enjoy and look forward to doing. If you can't find a physical activity you love to do, walk. The point is to do something.

You must be *consistent* and *diligent*.

If you have not exercised for years, please consult your doctor before beginning any new exercise regimen. Start out slowly. For instance, if you choose walking, walk for 10 minutes. When you feel that you have adjusted then add another 5 or 10 minutes. Keep adding minutes over a period of time. Soon you will have 30, 40, or 60 minutes of exercise.

Another way to approach the time factor is to break up your minutes over the course of a day. I've walked 15 minutes in the morning and then 15 minutes in the evening. Now, I walk 40 minutes a day, five days a week.

More Healthy Hints

- **Listen to your body.** If you experience pain or discomfort, STOP! See your doctor.

- **Change is good.** It's okay to change your exercise regimen. It allows you to work out different muscles.

- **Find a friend.** Sometimes it helps to exercise with someone. Make sure your support system speaks positive encouraging words.

- **Dress comfortably.** Wear clothing that allows you to breathe, maintain adequate circulation, and move freely. Choose appropriate fitness footwear that gives you the support you need to exercise effectively and prevent injury.

Prevention is Better Than a Cure

I feel anger and sadness when I see you lining the corridors of the E.R. or sitting in overcrowded physician's offices. Why? Because I know that a vast majority of sicknesses can be prevented. It is my heart's desire that you make a decision that will change your life for the better. Follow this biblically based road map to health and wellness. A new life awaits you! Embrace it today!

"Before I was afflicted
and went astray, but now
I keep Your word.

You are good and do good;
teach me Your statues."

Psalms 119: 67-68 58:11 NIV

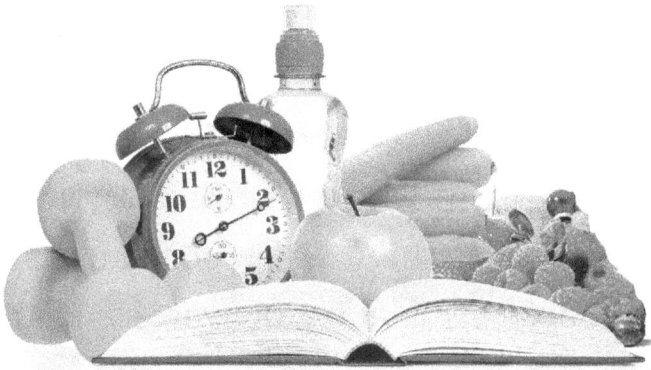

Chapter Five

Toxins and Waste

Toxin: *a poisonous substance and especially one that is produced by a living thing.*[1]

Waste: *loss of something valuable that occurs because too much of it is being used or because it is being used in a way that is not necessary or effective.*[2]

---

1. "Toxin." Merriam-Webster.com. 2011. http://www.merriamwebster.com (Retrieved August 2015).
2. "Waste." Merriam-Webster.com. 2011. http://www.merriamwebster.com (Retrieved August 2015).

I have saved this chapter for last. No one wants to talk about this subject. Yet, I believe that it is one of the most important chapters in this book. Elimination of waste and toxins is so important in helping our bodies maintain balance and health. We eliminate through our skin by sweating, through our kidneys with urination, and through our colon through bowel movements.

I heard about a surgeon who did exploratory surgery on a young man's bowel. The patient presented with a history of abdominal fullness, generalized fatigue, irritability, and bowel irregularities. The surgeon found a hard, black/green wad of stringy "junk." When they sent it to be analyzed it was undigested meat, that had been in the colon for at least 6 months. No wonder, this young man was so sick. Poor elimination, I believe, contributes to putting us at risk for sickness and disease.

So, let's be kind to our bodies, and keep our elimination systems clean. Drinking water allows toxins and waste to be removed. Remember, when your mother or grandmother would give you castor oil whenever the seasons changed? Well, in their wisdom, they were helping clean out your colon.

Another simple way to obtain this is to eat raw vegetables and fruits for a week or two. This will also help transition you into eating fresh veggies and fruits as a part of your everyday diet. To cleanse your bloodstream and detoxify, you can drink the juice of a fresh lemon in a warm 8 oz. glass of water in the morning and evening.

Let's be *kind* to our *bodies* and *keep* our elimination systems *clean!*

---

*"Don't you see that the
food you put into your body
cannot defile you? Food
doesn't go into your heart,
but only passes through the
stomach and then goes into
the sewer." And then He
added, "It is what comes from
inside that defiles you."*

Mark 7:18-20 NLT

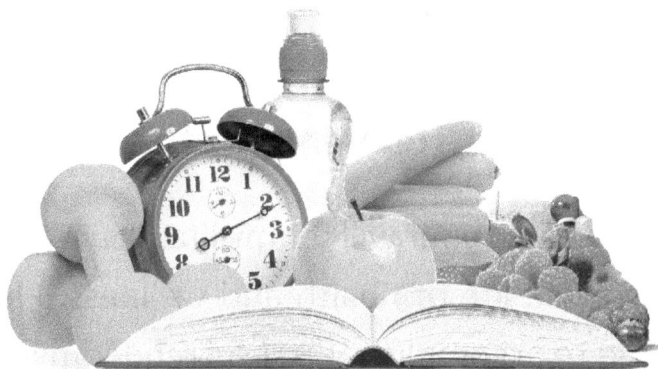

Chapter Six

A Prayer for a Health and Wellness Lifestyle

"I will answer them before they even call to me. While they are still talking about their needs, I will go ahead and answer their prayers!

Isaiah 65:24 NLT

Dear Heavenly Father

I now know your will for my life. You want me to live a life of health and wellness. Please help me to accomplish this. I surrender my mind and body completely to you. Fill me with the knowledge and understanding that I need now. Cause me to desire this on an every day basis. Cause me to walk in this lifestyle every day. I no longer want to do things that are detrimental to my body. Thank You for Your grace in all areas of my life. In Jesus' Name I pray,

… AMEN.

"I thank you for answering my prayer and giving me victory!"

Psalm 118:20-22

About the Author

Cheryall Sparks, RN

a registered nurse with more than thirty years of experience, Cheryall Sparks has dedicated her life to health and wellness. Her passion for preventative medicine and nutrition drove her to study and discover Heaven's plan for wholeness—spirit, soul, and body.

Cheryall's desire for everyone to walk in the health God meant for them to enjoy and have the strength to reach their destiny challenged her to search out all God's Word offers for healing, health, and wholeness.

In September 2015, Cheryall Sparks completed Joan Hunter's Healing School in Tomball, Texas, satisfied all the appropriate requirements and was ordained into the healing ministry under the covering of Joan Hunter Ministries and the 4 Corners Alliance.

Cheryall continues her work as a nurse as she steps fully into her calling. **Sick of Sick—Healthy Hints from Heaven** represents obedience to the assignment God gave her. He wants you to be healthy ... and Cheryall does too!

To learn more Healthy Hints or to invite
Cheryall to speak at your conference
or to your group contact:

HEALTHY HINTS from *Heaven,* LLC

P.O. Box 270834

Houston, TX 77277

832.781.8174

info@healthyhintsfromheaven.com

HEALTHY HINTS from *Heaven* LLC

P.O. Box 270834
Houston, TX 77277

832.781.8174
cheryall@yahoo.com

Promoting *health* and *wellness* God's way!

CHERYALL SPARKS, RN
President

DISCLAIMER

This book is based on the experiences, beliefs, and research of the author. All decisions regarding your health should be made with the approval of your health care provider. This book is intended to motivate and encourage the reader to make wise and healthy decisions. Use of the information contained in this book should be used with your own common sense and at your own risk. The material offered in this book is provided for general information purposes only and does not constitute professional medical or nutritional advice.

www.ingramcontent.com/pod-product-compliance
Lightning Source LLC
Chambersburg PA
CBHW060641280326
41933CB00012B/2105